"I Forgot You,
Please Don't Forget Me"
(If I Couldn't Laugh, I Would Be Crying)

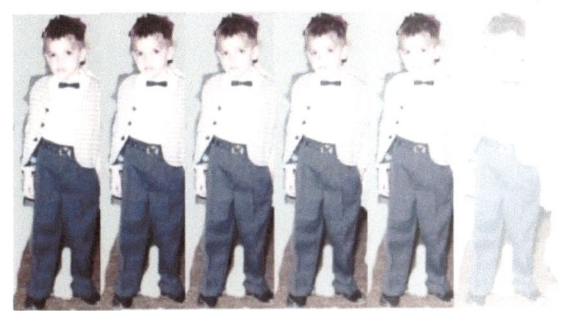

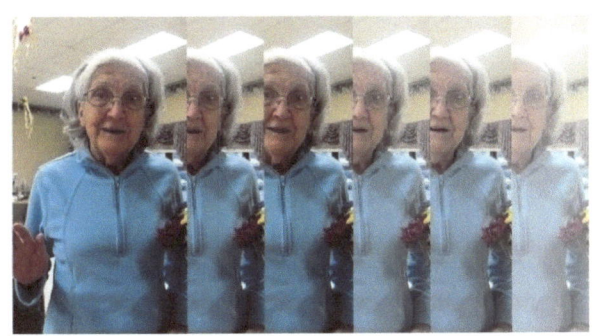

A Journey With Anna Through Alzheimer's

By John J. Gruba

ISBN-10: 1502997177
ISBN-13: 978-1502997173

Make me an instrument of peace.
That where there is hatred, let me bring love.
Where there is injury, may I bring pardon.
Where there is discord, may I bring harmony,
And where there is doubt, faith.
Where there is despair, may I bring hope.
Where there are shadows, may I bring light
And where there is sadness, may I bring joy.
Grant that I may offer comfort
Rather than seek to be comforted.
Grant also that I may understand
Rather than seek to be understood.
And grant I may give love,
Rather than seek to be loved.
For it is in giving that we receive.
It is by forgiving that we are forgiven.
God grant me the serenity to accept the things
I cannot change.
Courage to change the things I can
and the wisdom to know the difference.

After reading the

the sentence, you are

now aware that the

*the human brain often does not
inform you that the*

the word "the" has been

repeated twice every time.

Unknown

What is the difference between Alzheimer's and dementia?

Too often, patients and their family members are told by their doctors that the patient has been diagnosed with "a little bit of dementia." They leave the doctor's visit with a feeling of relief that at least they don't have Alzheimer's disease (AD). There is great confusion about the difference between dementia and Alzheimer's. The confusion is felt on the part of patients, family members, the media, and even healthcare providers. This article provides information to reduce the confusion by defining and describing these two common and often poorly understood terms.

"Dementia" is a term that has replaced a more out-of-date word, "senility," to refer to cognitive changes with advanced age. Dementia includes a group of symptoms, the most prominent of which is memory difficulty with additional problems in at least one other area of cognitive functioning, including language, attention, problem solving, spatial skills, judgment, planning, or organization. These cognitive problems are a noticeable change compared to the person's cognitive functioning earlier in life and are severe enough to get in the way of normal daily living, such as social and occupational activities.

A good analogy to the term dementia is "fever." Fever refers to an elevated temperature, indicating that a person is sick. But it does not give any information about what is causing the sickness. In the same way, dementia means that there is something wrong with a person's brain, but it does not provide any information about what is causing the memory or cognitive difficulties. Approximately 5.3 million Americans currently live with Alzheimer's disease. It is important to note, however, that although AD is extremely common in later years of life, it is not part of normal aging. For that matter, dementia is not part of normal aging.

If someone has dementia (due to whatever underlying cause), it represents an important problem in need of appropriate diagnosis and treatment by a well-trained healthcare provider who specializes in degenerative diseases. In a nutshell, dementia is a symptom, and Alzheimer's disease is the cause of the symptom. Contrary to what some people may think, dementia is not a less severe problem, with AD being a more severe problem.

There is not a continuum with dementia on one side and AD at the extreme. Rather, there can be early or mild stages of AD, which then progress to moderate and severe stages of the disease.

One reason for the confusion about dementia and AD is that it is not possible to diagnose AD with 100% accuracy while someone is alive. Rather, AD can only truly be diagnosed after death, upon autopsy when the brain tissue is carefully examined by a specialized doctor referred to as a neuropathologist.

And with the results of exciting new research, such as that being conducted at the BU ADC, the accuracy of AD diagnosis during life is getting better and better.

This contribution was made by Dr. Robert Stern, Director of the BU ADC Clinical Core. (Source Boston University Alzheimer's Disease Center Bulletin)

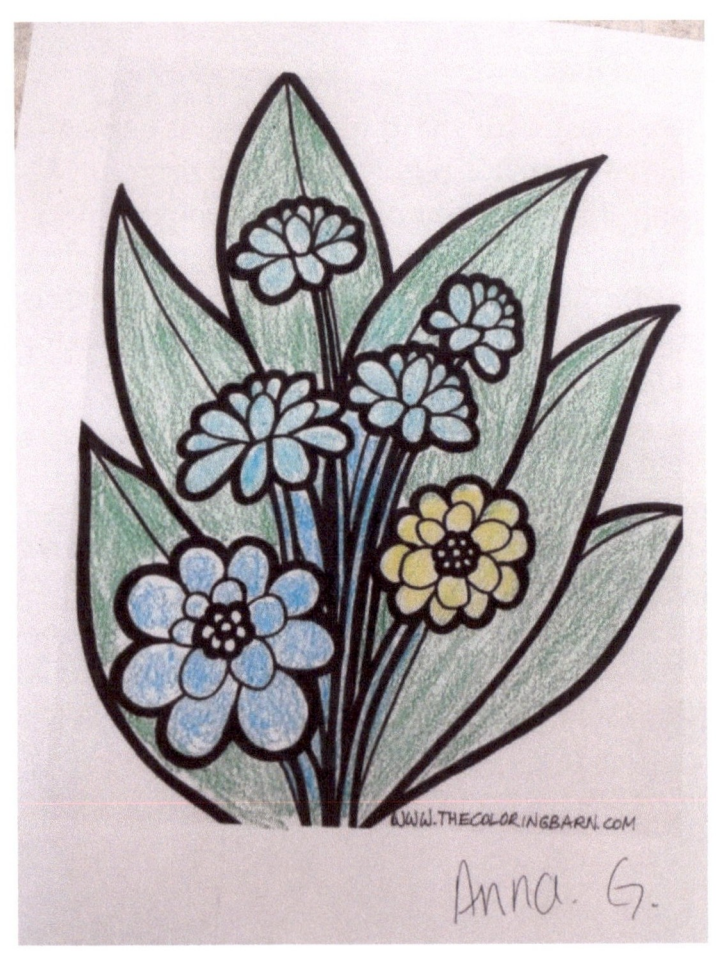

WWW.THECOLORINGBARN.COM

Anna. G.

I hope these will be helpful to you in visiting your loved one and enriching the time you have together. Written by Marie Marley is the award-winning author of Come Back Early Today: A Memoir of Love, Alzheimer's

Five of the most basic ones here: 1) Don't tell them they are wrong about something, 2) Don't argue with them, 3) Don't ask if they remember something, 4) Don't remind them that their spouse, parent or other loved one is dead, and 5) Don't bring up topics that may upset them.

Don't Tell Them They're Wrong About Something: To let the person save face, it's best not to contradict or correct them if they say something wrong. There's no good reason to do that. If they're alert enough, they'll realize they made a mistake and feel bad about it. Even if they don't understand their error, correcting them may embarrass or be otherwise unpleasant for them.

Don't Argue With the Person: It's never a good idea to argue with a person who has dementia. First of all, you can't win. And second, it will probably upset them or even make them angry. I learned a long time ago, when caring for my beloved Romanian soul mate, Ed, the best thing to do is simply change the subject -- preferably to something pleasant that will immediately catch their attention. That way, they'll likely forget all about the disagreement.

Don't Ask If They Remember Something: When talking with a person who has Alzheimer's, it's so tempting to ask them if they remember some person or event. "What did you have for lunch?" "What did you do this morning?" "Do you remember that we had candy bars when I visited last week?" "This is David. Do you remember him?" Of course they don't remember. Otherwise, they wouldn't have a diagnosis of dementia. It could embarrass or frustrate them if they don't remember. It's better to say, "I remember that we had candy the last time I was here. It was delicious."

Don't Remind the Person that a Loved One Is Dead: It's not uncommon for people with dementia to believe their deceased spouse, parent or other loved one is still alive. They may be confused or feel hurt that the person doesn't come to visit. If you inform them that the person is dead, they might not believe it and become angry with you. If they do believe you they'll probably be very upset by the news.

What's more, they're likely to soon forget what you said and go back to believing their loved one is still alive. An exception to this guideline is if they ask you if the person is gone. Then it's wise to give them an honest answer, even if they will soon forget it, and then go on to some other topic.

Don't Bring up Other Topics That May Upset Them: There's no reason to bring up topics you know may upset your loved one. If you don't see eye-to eye on politics, for example, don't even bring it up. It may just kindle an argument, which goes again the second guideline above. You won't prevail and it's just likely to cause them anger and/or frustration.

de·men·tia di-ˈmen(t)-shə: a mental illness that causes someone to be unable to think clearly or to understand what is real and what is not real

I had my first experience of a neurological disorder with my father-in-law, Roger. He was a hard working man who loved the country. He had a beautiful 5 acre horse farm where he and his wife lived for many years. When he was getting close to retirement, he and his wife bought a house in a small town down in the southern part of the state where they planned to retire. The company he was working for downsized and let him go sooner than he had planned. They sold the farm and moved. Up until then, he was a very active. He always had projects going on that kept him busy. In their new home, once they settled in, there were no projects, nothing really to keep him active, other than cutting the lawn, and that was his wife's job. So he sat on the porch and watched the grass grow. With nothing to do, no real purpose in life, he began to slip, mentally and physically. We found out later that his wife kept notes on his behavior and spoke to the doctor. I am pretty sure she had an idea of what was going on, but didn't share it with the family.

Roger had gotten sick and needed surgery. After that, his wife wasn't able to care for him, so she moved him to a local nursing home. The nursing home was understaffed and he wasn't able to get the rehabilitation services that he needed. My wife and I had taken the five hour drive to see him a couple of times. When we didn't see any improvement in his health, my wife offered to move him to a facility near us. It was a hard decision for his wife, but she realized it would be in his best interest. The first week or so was a little difficult for him, but having someone from his family visit every day helped with the adjustment. He was now getting the care and therapy he needed.

What is real, what is not real, this is dementia.

I visit Roger and bring along books on horses. He always knew the exact breeds and could tell you all about them. On one occasion we were sitting in his room talking about horses. I could see in his eyes that his mind was traveling somewhere else. He looked around the room and turned to me and said, "This is a real nice barn. You see how clean they keep it." What do you say? Do you tell him that he is in a nursing facility or do you go along for the ride. Of course, you go along for the ride.

There were times that he was confused who people were. Sometimes he thought my wife, his daughter, was his wife (that's confusing). He knew names and recognized faces, but couldn't connect relationships. If you asked him who Laurie was, he would say, "that's my wife".

Sometimes when we sat outside, he thought that he was living in a hotel; a hotel that the family owned. He remarked what a good job the employees were doing on keeping the place looking good. As a side note, the nursing facility was previously a hotel. So he wasn't that far off.

He loved westerns. The one thing that he never forgot was his John Wayne movies or the actors in them. Every night he had to watch a movie or two before going to bed.

As time went on, he began talking about his dad and his mom, more often. They had both passed long ago. He would tell us how he saw them and they were doing fine. We knew this was a sign that he was ready to leave us and join his parents.

He passed away very peacefully. My wife was with him. I prepared a beautiful funeral service for Roger. Everyone in the family was there. We cried, we laughed, and we told our stories about Roger. We celebrated his life.

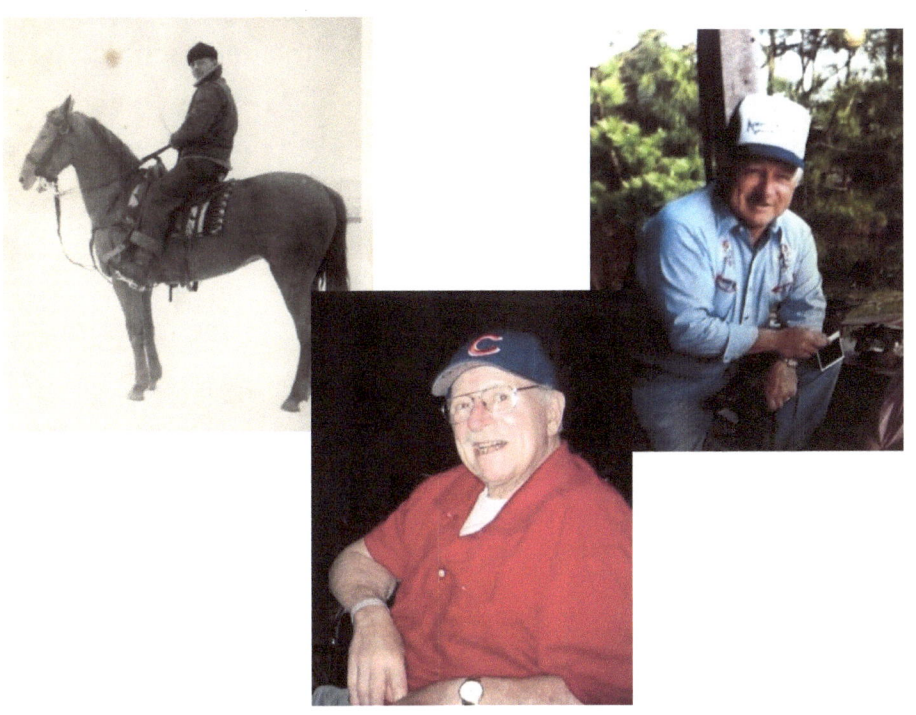

Alz·hei·mer's disease 'älts-ˌhī-mərz : a disease of the brain that causes people to slowly lose their memory and mental abilities as they grow old

In 2003 is when I began to notice that something wasn't quite right with my mother. She came to stay with us for 7 months, during her recovery from a broken arm; her second broken arm within a few years. This should have been an indication that something was wrong. Within a few years she managed to fall three times causing injury to herself. But she couldn't remember what caused her to fall.

She was lived alone in a third floor apartment. I wanted to find her an apartment closer to where I lived to keep an eye on her. I talked to her about moving. Some days she was ok with it. Other times she would say that she wanted to go back home. My brothers didn't think we should take away her independence. So, back she went back to her third floor apartment. Within the year she had fallen again. This time she fractured her pelvis. That's when it was decided by my brothers that assisted living is the place she needed to be. I didn't agree, but thought this was better than her living alone.

She lived at the assisted care facility for three years. Her activities included: hoarding paper, napkins, newspaper and bulletins, not taking her medication (putting her pills in a cup and hiding them in a cabinet), throwing away her laundry, and not showering. I visited her every other weekend, throwing out three or four bags of papers each time. Does this seem normal to you?

My mother, or Anna, suffers from Alzheimer's. She was medically diagnosed in 2008.

This is my definition of Alzheimer's and dementia – When people had a hard life, lived alone for a long time, and suffered from depression or anxiety, they exit from that life. They slowly let their memories go.

I moved her to a nursing home close to my house, actually in walking distance, when she fell and fractured her hip at the assisted care facility.

Bt this time, it was apparent that Mom had no short term memory. When we relocated her to the nursing facility, it threw her for a loop. She was disorientated. We had to remind her of her room number. She still asks me this almost every day. "What room am I in?" She had the same roommate, Millie, for almost two years. Mom couldn't remember that Millie was her roommate or Millie's name.

Just a side note: We were blessed that Millie was Mom's roommate. Millie was partially blind and 92 years young. She had all her faculties and watched out for Mom. Millie would make sure the CNAs dressed her properly and took her to all activities. It is with much sadness that Millie past away. We miss her.

Mom's long term memory is now going quickly. She doesn't recognize family members in pictures. Memory of my father has faded. Mom does not even recognize herself in pictures. I asked her if I can take a picture of her. "Are you are taking a picture of me with a phone?"

"Yes, Anna, this is my phone." She was puzzled. I can hear her thoughts, "This guy is taking a picture of me with a phone and they tell me I have Alzheimer's'."

I show her the photo and she says, "Who is that?" "It's you", I say. "That's not me. That person is old." I think that people with Alzheimer's and dementia see themselves as young people. People with Alzheimer's and dementia are like kids, we have to make sure they eat, use the fork and knife, make sure they go to the washroom, use a Kleenex and you pay attention.

Mom has checked out, but my friend, Anna stepped in. Anna has brought humor to an ungodly disease.

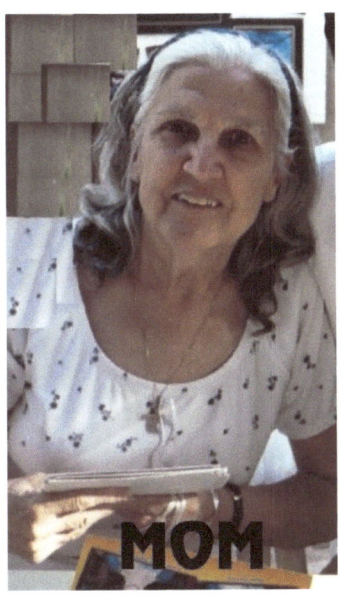 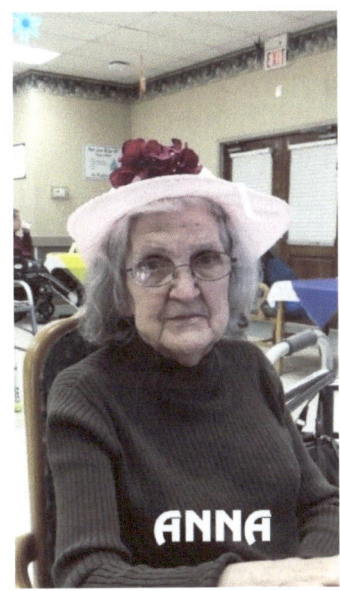

Is that my car over there?

My mother was in a very bad car accident when she was 17. Ever since then, she has been afraid of getting behind the wheel. I remember one winter when I was a kid and my father got the car stuck in snow. He asked my mother to get behind the wheel and give it some gas. She refused. Needless to say we left the car where it was stuck in the snow.

When my mother arrived at the nursing residence, after her hip surgery, she was in a wheel chair. Every time we started walking, she would say, "Does this (the wheelchair) go with me?" She learned how to use the wheelchair like an expert. Part of her therapy at meal time would be for a CNA to get her out of the wheelchair and walk her into the dining room.

One day, after lunch, she said, "Do you know where my car is?"

"Mom you started driving?", I asked.

"Oh it's over there." She points to the wheel chair. She asked me, "Where is your car?"

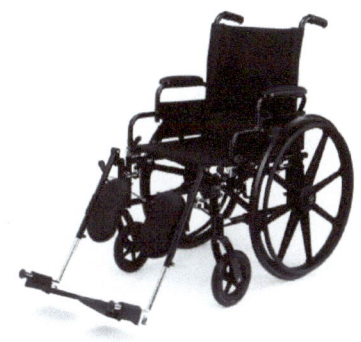

Mom's Car

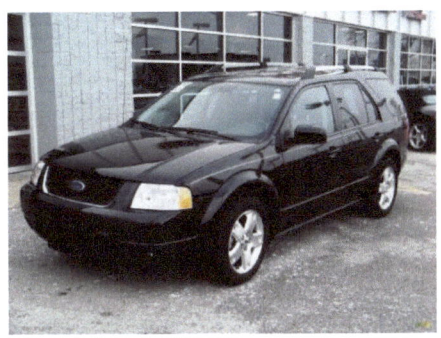

My Car

They are both the same color.

Can you tell the kids to behave?

This picture is hanging up at the residence.

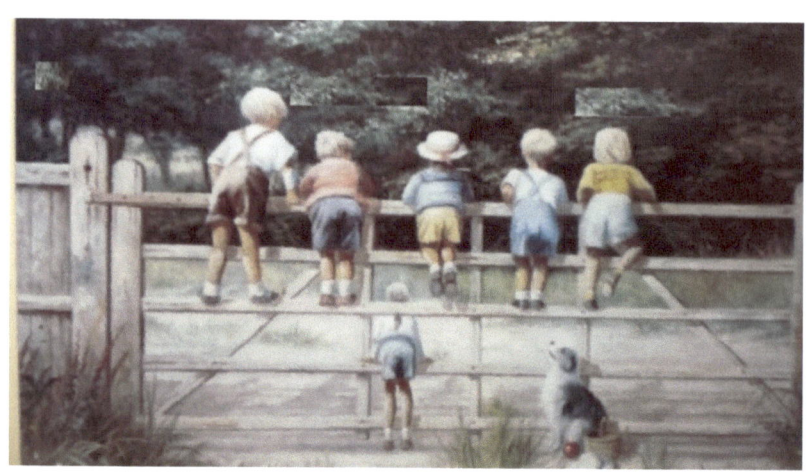

Mom said, "You see those kids?

Yesterday they were facing the other way."

Nest? Shoes?

Every nursing facility I've been in has a finch aviary. Mom was looking at the aviary and said, "Don't those things (nests) look like baby shoes."

"Well, you know the other day, someone opened the cage and put them on like shoes. They were running around."

I thought to myself, "It was probably you."

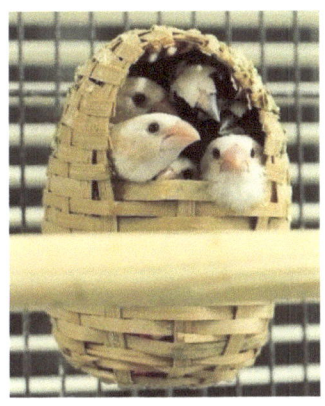 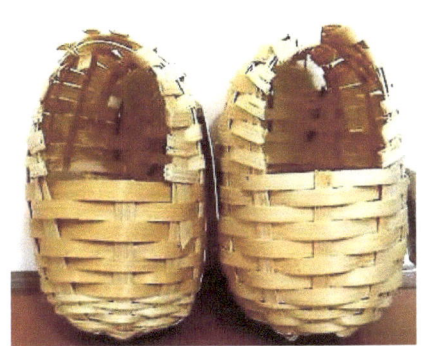

Nest   or   Shoes

My mother's life...in her own words.

Mom was sitting outside one day with Millie and Millie's son George. Mom told them about her trips to Sicily. That sparked her to tell how she came over here, to the USA, as a little girl from Sicily. She couldn't speak English, only Italian, and it was hard, but she mastered the language.

George was very impressed. The next time I saw him, he told me what Mom had said about coming from another country. I looked at him a little surprised. I asked George if the she said the country she came from was Chicago and the boat she took was on Lake Michigan.

Mom: You know they call me by the wrong name around here.

Me: What is your name?

Mom: Anna Zonzo

Me: What name do they call you?

Mom: Anna Gruba

Me: You were married, Mom, to John Gruba.

(She thinks and shakes her head no)

Me: John Gruba?

Mom: You're John Gruba. (Pause) Are you my husband?

Me: No, I am your son. (She looks at me perplexed.)

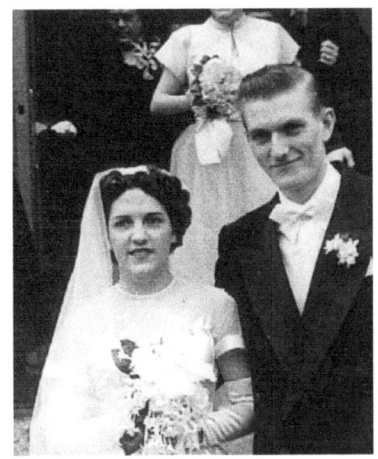 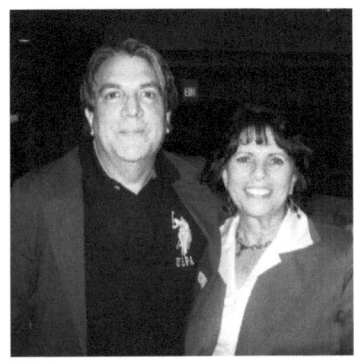

John Gruba   or   **John Gruba**

Next Round

Me: Did you have a boyfriend at the last place you lived at?

Mom: After five husbands who wants another man.

Me: (I'm perplexed) What was your last husband's name?

Mom: Giuseppe. If you're my son, which number are you?

Me: Number three.

Mom: That's right. Joseph is after you.

Me: (In my head) Joseph? Who's Joseph? I am still trying to figure out who Dominic is.

Seeing people change
Isn't what hurts

What hurts is remembering who they
used to be

This Was Mom's Real Life

My mother was born in Chicago, in the Logan Square neighborhood.

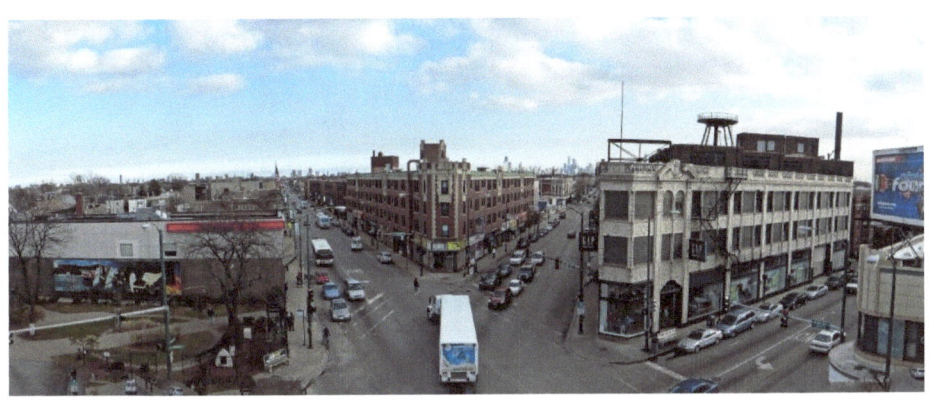

This was my mom's favorite area. We used to call it "down the avenue". Shopping, Movie Theater, Restaurants. Mom used to go out at least 3 times a day. She would meet friends and socialize, get the latest gossip.

From the age of 12, she lived in this apartment building. She lived on the third floor for 50 years. Her Mom and older sister lived on the first floor, her younger sister lived on the second floor.

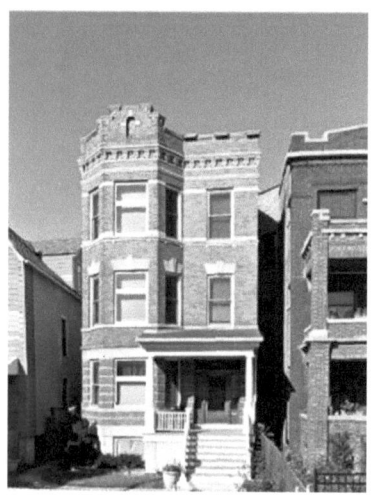

Her mother and father came from Italy.

Mom's maiden name is Zonzo. Her married name is Gruba. She was married to John Gruba; they separated after 25 years. He passed away at the age of 53 in 1984.

She has four sons. No one named Joseph. But, her grandfather's name was Joseph.

DO NOT ASK ME TO REMEMBER,
DON'T TRY TO MAKE ME UNDERSTAND.
LET ME REST
AND KNOW YOU'RE WITH ME,
KISS MY CHEEK AND HOLD MY HAND.
I'M SO CONFUSED
BEYOND YOUR CONCEPT,
I AM SAD AND SICK AND LOST.
ALL I KNOW IS THAT I NEED YOU,
TO BE WITH ME AT ALL COST.
SO DO NOT LOSE
YOUR PATIENCE WITH ME,
DO NOT SCOLD OR CURSE OR CRY.
I CAN'T HELP THE WAY I'M ACTING,
CAN'T BE DIFFERENT THOUGH I TRY.
JUST REMEMBER THAT I NEED YOU,
THAT THE BEST OF ME IS GONE.
PLEASE DON'T FAIL
TO STAND BESIDE ME,
LOVE ME 'TIL MY LIFE IS GONE.

Unknown

Boys? Girls?

Mom is at the point where she knows my name, but doesn't acknowledge that I'm her son. However, all the other women at the nursing facility think I'm their son.

One day I went to see her. I was also there the day before. She said, "Hi, I haven't seen you in a long time."

I replied, "Maybe a few years?"

She smiled.

Her CNA said, "Anna are you glad that your son is here?"

"I don't have sons. I have all girls," she replied.

Really confusing. I didn't want to go there.

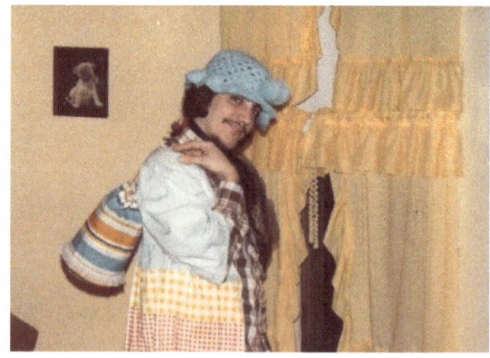

Kids that don't grow up

There is no time continuum with Alzheimer's patients. We brought Mom to the house for lunch one day. While we were sitting in the living room she heard someone upstairs.

"Who's upstairs?" she asked.

I said, "It's Gabriel, my son". She asked if she could see him. I called him downstairs and he greeted his grandmother. As he walked away she said, "That's not Gabriel". (Me) "Yes it is". (Mom) "He is supposed to be a little boy".

Gabriel went back upstairs. About an hour later she wants to know who's upstairs. Gabriel was coming down the stairs again and she asked him, "Who are you?" "I am Elvis." Mom said, "Okay Elvis".

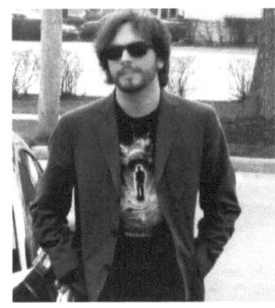 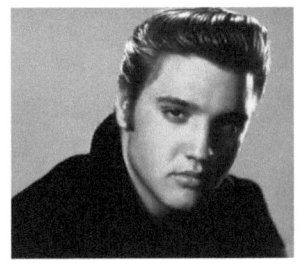

I think he is Elvis's clone

Do you know the secret hand symbol for coffee?

My mother loved coffee. Any where she went she would always ask for a cup of coffee.

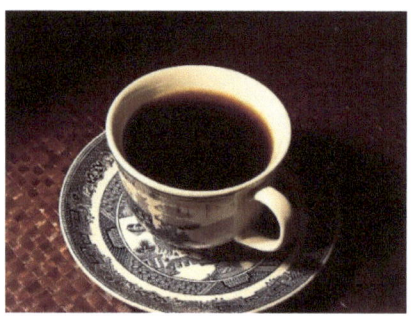

She created her own symbol for a cup of coffee. We have been using it for years. She would always say, "I would like a good cup of coffee" or "Are you making coffee?"

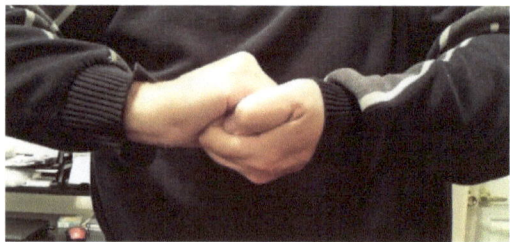

THE SECRET HAND SYMBOL FOR COFFE

Now, it's not about the coffee. At the nursing facility at mealtime they would not let her have coffee until she was 75% done eating her food. If she gets the coffee first, she barely eats anything.

Lately, she has no interest or need for food or coffee. When she sits down to eat, with her pureed food, (she threw out her teeth the second week she was at the nursing facility) she swirls the food around on the dish and re-arranges it in piles according to color and height. The she asks, "Does this look okay?"

I am ready for my close up Mr. DeMille

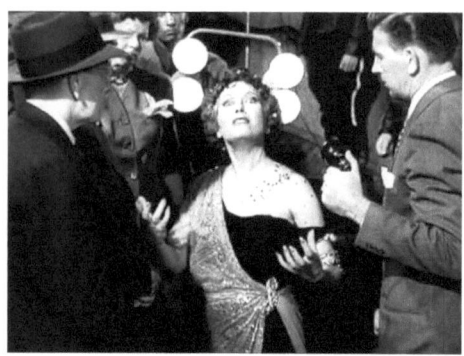

What is vanity? The dictionary tells us it is excessive pride in one's appearance. What is obsessive? The dictionary tells us it is being continually preoccupied with a particular activity, person, or thing. I put the two definitions together and I get Anna.

Mom was always worried about her appearance. I guess that sometimes if you don't have money, but you are around people that do, you sometimes may think you need what they have. And, if you don't have it, you worry about how you fit in. To some people, it is not what's inside that counts, but what is on the outside. And, over the years this may become an obsession, maybe more than just vanity for Mom.

There were also those who would buy her clothes when she was down and out. I'm not talking about every day clothes, but clothes you'd wear to fancy parties or places. Of course, she rarely did that, but the expensive clothes made her feel good.

Mom is still constantly worried about her appearance. She asks everyone about how she looks. Every mirror, or every reflection she comes across, she has to look at herself. She stops and fixes her hair and turns to whoever is with her and says, "How does this look?" When she gets up out of a chair she brushes her butt, fixes her top, and fixes her crotch, just like a baseball player, right there in the open, with everyone watching. She turns to anyone looking at her and says, "How do I look? Is my back straight? Do my pants look okay?"

Some days this goes on for hours. Does my top look okay? Yes, Mom. She adjusts her top. How is this? One of the aides once asked her, "How does my back look?" My mom, I mean Anna, took the aide's smock and straightened it and said; "Now it looks good."

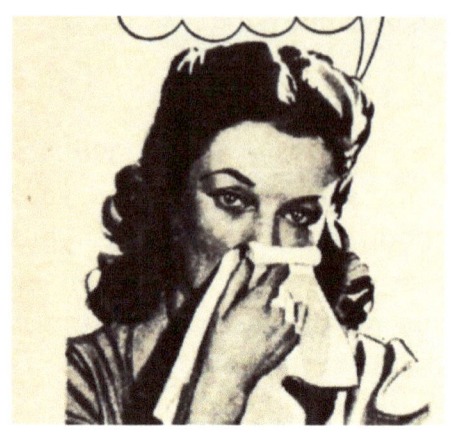

"Can you get me a Kleenex for my nose", Mom says. She always thinks her nose is running and there, hidden and overflowing from her sleeve, is a Kleenex. She takes one and gently touches her nose, inhales twice and then wipes the table off with the Kleenex.

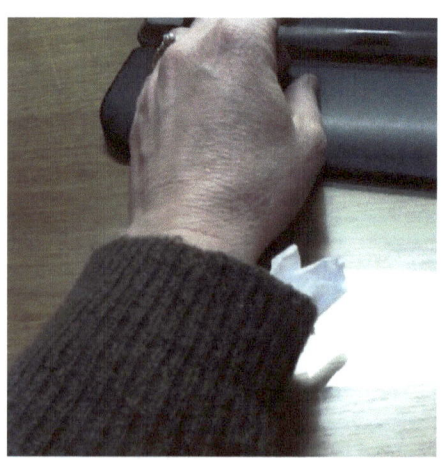

What number did they call?

Monday afternoons and Thursday mornings are BINGO at the nursing facility. This helps the residents recognize numbers and letters. Most of the residents are capable of playing, but there are some that need a little help. Mom is a very vigilant bingo player. When a number is called, like N34, chip in her hand, she goes right down the N list.

B	I	N	G	O
14	20	32	52	71
10	27	42	55	64
7	23	FREE	58	69
11	28	34	56	72
15	25	33	53	66

I go on Monday afternoons to help out and socialize with the other visitors. I walk in and there's Mom waving her arms as if she is drowning, calling, "John. John. I have to tell you something".

I say my hellos to all the residents and make my way over to Mom. The first question Mom asks, "Do I look okay?" And before I could answer, "How does my hair look? What about my back?"

I began to notice that she was asking several questions about bingo after my arrival. "What number did they call? What am I suppose to do with these things (the chips)? What do they mean by B?" The list goes on.

It took me a couple of weeks to figure out what she was doing. Before I got there, the aide said she is playing fine by herself. The answer is "jealousy". There are four residents to a table. I usually have people sit next to me who need help because they can't physically put the chips on the numbers or they don't understand what is going on. At this point I am not paying a lot of attention to her. As I am talking or taking care of the other person, Mom will tap my arm and just talk away, saying my name about 50 times. "John. John."

I never get mad and I try, I mean really try, to be patient. My father used to say "Patience is a virtue." He didn't have this virtue, and neither do I, but I am learning.

Other things that drive me crazy

Residents are served snacks in the afternoon around 3:00 pm. Mom gets pudding or ice cream or something pureed because she doesn't have teeth (she threw them out) and pockets her food like a hamster. We go through a daily routine of:

Mom: "Whose is this?"

Me: "That's yours, Mom".

Mom: "Is it on the table okay?", as she moves it and her napkin. "How does this look? Is it okay?"

Me: "Yes, Mom, eat your pudding". I turn around to talk to somebody and there she is, licking the pudding out of the container. "Mom could you please use your spoon".

Mom: "It is right here," (the spoon is on the table).

Me: "Do you want to go back to your room?"

Mom: "What room?"

Me: "Your room. Number 10".

Mom: "What is your room number?"

Me: "Mom, I don't live here". And then we go through where I live and I tell her I have a wife and kids.

Mom: "You're married. No one told me." "Do you have a walker? Somebody must have poured water on this chair because my pants are wet."

Take a deep breath and count to 10.

1 2 3 4 5 6 7 8 9 10

There is a Surprise

I am always surprised that within the realm of Mom's Alzheimer's she has no problem doing word searches. Forward, backwards, diagonal. Also we play fill in the blanks. I write down some letters and she tells me what is missing.

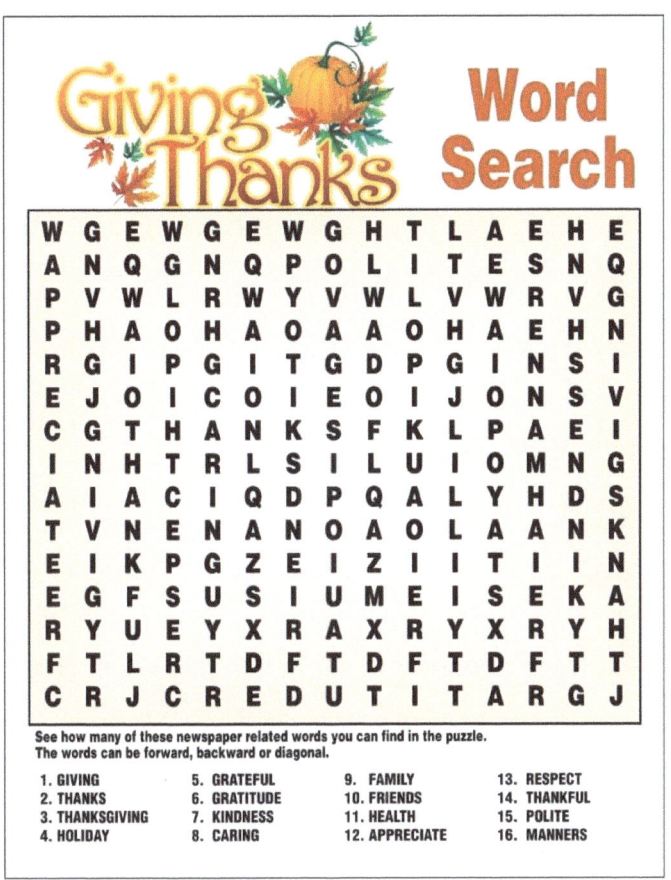

I have found the one in a million

Alzheimer's is a long hard journey. And finding a place for a loved one with dementia or Alzheimer's is a difficult task. When Laurie and I set out on finding a home for Roger we began by going to visit all the nursing facilities in the area.

This was our checklist:

Check with the state to see how they rate and how many complaints they have. Were the complaints resolved?

First Impressions on the phone – Was the person who answered courteous – Did they seem informative

Outside Appearance – was the property kept clean, flowers, shrubs, or trees. Was there somewhere for the residents to sit outside - Was there anybody outside the day we visited.

Walking In – Did we have to ring a bell to get in (security) - Did someone greet us immediately - Did it smell (Three of the places did.)

Inside – Did we see people interacting with the residents – Did the rooms look clean – If it was lunchtime were the residents being taken care of – Did a staff member show you the rooms (including the therapy room)

Think about if you felt good about the staff you talked to – Do you feel that your loved one would be secure – Did the home offer to help you with all the paperwork (there is a lot of it) – What about your questions such as public aid, who is the doctor, what happens if they have to go the hospital – What do they have for activities.

We chose Heritage Health for Roger. The two years he was there, we met some great workers, from activities, housekeeping, kitchen staff, administration, the nurses and of course, the soldiers, CNAs (Certified Nursing Assistants). Heritage has a very low turnover for CNAs. Can you imagine taking care of more than one person with Alzheimer's or dementia? What about bathing? What about going to the washroom or changing their soiled clothes? It takes very special people to do all this. This is why I have Heritage Health taking care of my Mom. They helped me out with all the paperwork, including public aid. They honor my wishes for Mom to go to all the activities, even when I am not there. I have a great friendship with all the employees. There are a few who are my favorites. If I have any complaints they listen to me and we resolve them before they become a problem.

Really do your homework. Ask every question you can think of (even the minor ones). All questions should be answered.

Heritage Health, in the northwest suburbs of Chicago, is the place where I know that Mom is getting the great care and staying active.

Each Alzheimer's caregiver needs to come to a simple understanding –

Your accomplishment is wonderful and amazing.

Bob DeMarco, Founder
AlzheimersReadingRoom.com

BLESSED ARE THEY
WHO UNDERSTAND

We can't change the past. Of course hindsight is 20/20. We have to move forward and not dwell on what could have been. We were dysfunctional before the word was coined. We thought we were normal. Out to dinner meant going to the local bar, we got a hamburger and fries, Dad got the Old Style. All our close friends went out to dinner at the same bar.

Let the past go, we have all made mistakes, and look ahead to the lessons we learned.

Thank you for reading my journey with Anna. I hope it put a smile on your face. I can't change the disease, but I can make sure she is safe, healthy, and happy.

Though those with Alzheimer's might forget us,

We as a society must remember them.

-Scott Kirschenbaum-

Stages of Alzheimer's Disease

Experts have documented common patterns of symptom progression that occur in individuals with Alzheimer's disease. Based on these patterns, they developed several methods of "staging."

Alzheimer's disease advances at widely different rates. Not everyone will experience every symptom, and symptoms may occur at different times in different individuals. People with Alzheimer's live an average of eight years after diagnosis, but may survive anywhere from three to 20 years.

Determining which stage an individual has reached helps families and health care professionals make better care decisions. Individuals with the disease and their families can prepare themselves for the progression of the disease. People with dementia can get involved with clinical studies through Alzheimer's Association Trial Match®.

Staging the disease using the Global Deterioration Scale (GDS)

The Global Deterioration Scale is a system that outlines key symptoms and is characterized by seven stages ranging from unimpaired function to very severe cognitive decline.

NOTE: GDS stages correspond to the widely used concepts of mild, moderate, moderately severe and severe Alzheimer's disease. Also noted are which stages fall within the more general divisions of early-stage, mid-stage and late-stage categories.

Stage 1 –Preclinical Stage

Description: A newly defined stage reflecting current evidence that measurable biomarker changes in the brain may occur years before symptoms affecting memory, thinking or behavior can be detected by affected individuals or their physicians. While the guidelines identify these preclinical changes as an Alzheimer's stage, they do not establish diagnostic criteria that doctors can use now. Rather, they propose additional research to establish which biomarkers may best confirm that Alzheimer's-related changes are under way and how to measure them.

Symptoms: No impairment (normal function). No experience with memory problems. An interview with a medical professional does not show any evidence of dementia symptoms.

Stage 2 –Early Stage

Description: Mild cognitive decline. Difficulty in social or occupational settings.

Friends or family may notice change.

Symptoms: Very mild cognitive decline (may be normal age-related changes or earliest signs of Alzheimer's disease). The person may experience memory lapses—forgetting familiar words or the location of everyday objects —but no symptoms of dementia can be detected during a medical examination or by friends, family or co-workers.

Stage 3 –Early Stage

Description: Mild cognitive impairment (MCI) due to Alzheimer's disease. In this stage, mild changes in memory and thinking are noticeable and can be measured on mental status tests, but are not severe enough to disrupt day-to-day life.

Symptoms: Mild cognitive decline. Friends, family or co-workers begin to notice difficulties. During a detailed medical interview, doctors may be able to detect problems in memory or concentration.

Common stage 3 difficulties include:

Noticeable problems coming up with the right word or name.

Trouble remembering names when introduced to new people.

Experiencing noticeably greater difficulty performing tasks in social or work settings.

Forgetting material that was just read.

Losing or misplacing valued objects.

Increasing trouble with planning or organizing

Stage 4 –Early Stage

Description: Probable Alzheimer's dementia. The differentiation of dementia from MCI rests on the determination of whether there is significant interference in the ability to function at work or in usual daily activities. This is a clinical judgment based on information obtained from the patient and from a knowledgeable informant.

Symptoms: Moderate cognitive decline (mild or early-stage Alzheimer's disease).At this point, a careful medical interview should be able to detect clear-cut symptoms in several areas:

Forgetfulness of recent events.

Impaired ability to perform challenging mental arithmetic —for example, counting backward from 00 by 7s.

Greater difficulty performing complex tasks, such as planning dinner for guests, paying bills or managing finances.

Forgetfulness about personal history.

Becoming moody or withdrawn, especially in socially or mentally challenging situations.

Stage 5 –Middle Stage

Description: Moderate cognitive decline. Difficulty performing simple tasks.

May need assistance with activities of daily living such as bathing or dressing.

Symptoms: Moderately severe cognitive decline (moderate or mid-stage Alzheimer's disease). Gaps in memory and thinking are noticeable ,and assistance with daily activities is needed.

At this stage, the following changes may occur: Inability to recall home address, telephone number, or the names of high school or colleges attended. Confusion about time or place.

Trouble with less challenging mental arithmetic; such as counting backward from 40 by subtracting 4s or from 20 by subtracting 2s.

Difficulty choosing proper clothing for the season or the occasion.

Significant details about one's self and family may still be recalled.

Assistance eating or using the toilet may be required.

Stage 6 –Middle Stage

Description: Severe cognitive decline.

Symptoms: Moderately severe or mid-stage Alzheimer's disease. Memory continues to worsen, personality changes may take place and extensive assistance is needed to complete activities of daily living.

At this stage, the following changes may occur:

Loss of awareness of recent experiences as well as surroundings.

No changes in ability to recall one's own name, but difficulty recalling personal history.

Ability to distinguish between familiar and unfamiliar faces continues, but there may be difficulty remembering the name of a spouse or caregiver.

Assistance to dress properly and avoid mistakes such as putting pajamas over daytime clothes or shoes on the wrong feet.

Major changes in sleep patterns, including sleeping during the day and becoming restless at night.

Help with handling details of toileting (flushing the toilet, wiping or disposing of tissue properly).

Increasingly frequent trouble controlling bladder or bowels.

Major personality and behavioral changes, including suspiciousness and delusions (such as believing that a caregiver is an impostor), or compulsive, repetitive behaviors (such as hand-wringing or tissue-shredding).

A tendency to wander or become lost.

Stage 7 –Late Stage

Description: Severe impairment. Supervision or complete assistance is required to complete all activities of daily living. Communication is severely impaired.

Symptoms: Very severe cognitive decline (severe or late-stage Alzheimer's disease).

In the final stage of this disease, losses include the ability to respond to the environment, carry on a conversation and, eventually, to control movement. Communication with words and phrases may be possible.

At this stage, assistance or supervision will be required to complete most daily personal care, including eating and using the toilet. Losses may include the ability to smile, sit without support and to hold one's head up. Reflexes become abnormal, muscles grow rigid and swallowing is impaired.

TS-0050 | Updated February 2014

alzheimer's ℚ℧ association®

the compassion to care, the leadership to conquer˙

About The Author

A dedicated professional, John J. Gruba is a self-employed certified Holistic Health Practitioner, who is deeply committed to sharing his passion for health and well-being with others. He has over 12 years of experience as a healer with a special focus on Aura/Chakra Analysis, Reiki, Past Lives and the Akashic Records. He is also trained in Oracle Card Reading, Soul Coaching, Chakra Therapy, and Emotional Freedom Technique. He has experience working with many different clients, children to the elderly.

Influenced by Jack Canfield, Doreen Virtue and Louise Hay, John is particularly grateful to Reverend James Kwasigroch, who taught him the importance of love, compassion and healing.

John is an Interfaith Minister with The Universal Church of the Divine. He was ordained Minister of Spiritual Studies at The National Interfaith Seminary and earned a bachelor's degree in Pastoral Counseling from the Interfaith Seminary in New Rochelle, NY. He is an Angel Therapy Practitioner certified by Doreen Virtue, PhD., and has taken additional post-education courses in reflexology and neuro linguistic programming.

John is the author of "I Forgot You, Please Don't Forget Me (If I Couldn't Laugh, I Would Be Crying)" a journey through Alzheimer's, "Start Shifting", all about affirmations and "The Akashic Records", a short lesson on the book of life.

Despite his busy career, John makes time to be involved with community and professional organizations. He is a member of the International Natural Healers Association and the World Metaphysical Association. He has volunteered for Hospice (Twilight Brigade) and is on the Resident and Family Council at Heritage Health Therapy & Senior Care.

John lives in the Northwest Suburbs of Chicago with his wife, Laurie.

Visit John's website at
www.revjgruba.webs.com

www.ingramcontent.com/pod-product-compliance
Lightning Source LLC
Chambersburg PA
CBHW050821290526
45792CB00001B/206